Eyelash Extension Tr[...]
Master The Eyelash Extension Tech[...] Your Skill

By Julia Broderick

Table Of Contents

Introduction

Chapter 1
All About Eyelash Extensions

Chapter 2
Types Of Lashes: Length, Thickness, Curl

Chapter 3
Application Tools and Products

Chapter 4
Hair Growth Cycle and Anatomy of Eyelashes

Chapter 5
Health & Safety

Chapter 6
Structures, Eye Shapes and Styles

Chapter 7
Preparation, Application and Removal

Chapter 8
Client Home Maintenance

Chapter 9
Marketing and Pricing

Introduction

It's a recent trend that shows no sign of slowing down. The reason for it's great increase in popularity, is because of it's innovative nature. In an era where less is more and where the natural look is how we like to roll when it comes to "getting dolled up," it only makes sense to highlight certain facial attributes in a more subtle, yet noticeable way. That's where eyelash extensions comes in. With a high demand, comes the potential for good business and eyelash extensions have favoured that potential. It has become quite the lucrative speciality in it's own right in the field of esthetics.

Salon owners are always on the lookout for technicians as the demand increases. Unfortunately, not many can do the job properly due to lack of proper training. This is what I have come to realize after years of working in the field, as a formally trained and working eyelash technician and trainer myself. The technique involved is a very precise and meticulous one, that demands patience on the technician's part.

Let's face it ladies, putting on mascara, let alone everything else, cuts into our beauty sleep. What would you think if I went as far as to tell you that some women say their lash extensions allow them to get away with using less makeup? Or that some are so impressed with their new look, that they just skip makeup altogether. It's true!

As a technician, you can charge big money for a first time set of lashes, we're talking anywhere between $100 to $300, depending on your city! Imagine earning what you would, if not more than a 9to5 without the 9to5.

So by the end of this book, you'll have learned:

-The theory and history of eyelash extensions

-Proper application and technique

-Types of eyelash extensions

-Anatomy of the lashes

-Correct posture

-Hand positioning

-Health and Safety

-Hygiene

-Proper customer service

-Home maintenance for the client

-Product knowledge

-Eyelash technician terminologies

-Styling, eye structures, eye shapes

-Business, marketing and how to grow your business

to name a few!

Believe it or not, eyelash extensions can not only accentuate your eyes but can also create the illusion of having completely transformed one's features (for the better of course). Long gone are the days of false strip lashes! Women can now wake up everyday with their own semi permanent beautiful long voluminous lashes.

Chapter 1

All About Eyelash Extensions

The eyelash extension technique actually originated in South Korea. What differentiates eyelash extensions from your typical false lashes (available at your local drug store; i.e. strip or cluster lashes) aside from their effect of course, is that lash extensions are single eyelashes derived either of real mink fur (which is not highly recommended) or synthetic materials such as faux mink and silk. The technique consists of gluing each individual extension one at a time to the natural lash. This is why the eyelash extensions fall when the natural lashes fall and why refills become necessary (just like we go for refills for our fake nails) after 2-4 weeks. The amount of time that the eyelashes last, depends on your client's hair growth cycle, your technique as the eyelash technician, the glue that you work with, climate and client home maintenance.

The first time process (full set) can take a new technician about 2 hours. A refill usually takes 30-45 minutes.

A client can really live a normal life after having their eyelash extensions done but always remind and inform your client that because glue is the bond that adheres the extension to their natural lash, they will need to keep from exposing their newly done lashes to wet environments, heat & humidity, (i.e. not spending an entire day sunbathing).

Over exposure can weaken the glue and cause the extensions to fall out prematurely. If a nano mister (more on tools and equipment in chapter 3) is not used in the session (to cure the glue immediately) or the glue is one that only requires a 24 to 48 hour drying time, then the client should avoid getting their lashes,wet for that said time.

The client can't wet their lashes, exercise, shower, go swimming, wear make-up, withstand vapour (i.e. sauna) or heat (i.e. sun bathing) for the required amount of time.

At all times **oils** are to be avoided, as well as mascara (especially waterproof).Clients need to use products that are either water based, or specifically designed for eyelash extensions.

Before starting a full set or refill session, technicians must always ensure that their client is not wearing any makeup or contacts. The length and thickness of the client's natural lash will serve as a reference point as to what type of extension (weight,length,thickness) to use.

Chapter 2

Types Of Lashes: Length, Thickness, Curl

Numerous variations of eyelash extensions are available in today's market. Faux eyelash extensions are made with synthetic fibres. Two of the more popular extensions used on the market are mink and silk lashes. Minks are the most popular material to work with and are meant to provide a feathery, light, natural look. Silk is meant for a more dramatic look and is darker than minks.

There are different lengths, curls and thicknesses on the market to choose from. The most popular lengths vary anywhere from 6-17 mm. As for thicknesses there are 0.10, 0.12, 0.15, 0.18, 0.20, 0.25, 0.30 for classic eyelash extensions (1 on 1 method which is what we are learning in this book). For curls, the basic curls that are used are *J,B,C,D,L.*

How to choose the proper length for your client:

You will need to measure the client's natural lash length by taking a 10mm lash extension and placing it near the client's real lash. If the client's lash is longer than the 10 mm, then you will need to estimate by eye, how many mm's longer it is and vice versa if the natural lash length is shorter than 10mm.

Once you've estimated the general size of the natural lash, you will need to add the number 3 to that length by doing simple math (example below). That number will determine the maximum length that you are permitted to use on that client to avoid damaging the lashes.

Example: You just measured Lina's lashes by placing a 10mm extension near her natural lash. 2 mm of her natural lashes surpassed the 10mm extension meaning her lashes measured 12mm.

10+2= 12

By adding 3 to the 12
 3+12=15mm

You know that you cannot place more than 15mm on her natural lashes although you can put less than 15mm if you choose to.

Note* You would not do this for every single individual eyelash. You will measure the longest lash one time. Whatever number you get after measuring and adding 3, will be considered the client's natural lash length.

How to choose the curl:

This is very simple. J curl does not have much of a curl to it, use it on someone who wants a natural look, on older women or someone who has very curled natural lashes. (Putting a curled extension on an already curled lash can look funny and will touch the skin of the eyelid).

Same goes for B's. B's have slightly more of a curl than J's but still not much of a curl to it.

C is the most popular one, has a great curl to it. Just right!

D is very curled and gives a dramatic doll like effect.

L is extremely curled up and is meant to really open up the eyes. The curlier the extension the more the eyes pop!

How to determine the thickness:

- 0.10mm is for thin lashes
- 0.15mm is for medium lashes
- 0.20mm is for thick lashes
- 0.12 is in between thin and medium
- 0 .18 is in between med and thick
- 0.25-0.30 is very thick and I would advise to stay away from those thicknesses to avoid damaging the natural lashes

You will eventually be able to tell the difference between thin, medium and thick lashes as you start to get more experience. For now, just place the thicknesses near the natural lashes and use the thickness that is closest to the natural lash as a guide).

Note* applying a lash that is too long and heavy for natural lashes can cause temporary to permanent damage and hair loss. Always respect the natural lashes to ensure the health and safety of your client's eyelashes.

Chapter 3

Application Tools and Products

Like any other craft, the practice of the eyelash extension technique is not without it's tools and respective purposes. In this chapter we will discuss the importance of the tools for application. There are many different gadgets and tools on the market. Here, we will discuss the necessary ones. The right tools can make all the difference. Please make sure to use quality products from reputable suppliers, as this could make all the difference in your work. A good quality glue will ensure great results and bonding power as well quality lashes will make them look amazing.

- Straight tweezers: this is the tweezer that you will use to grab your eyelash extension with your dominant hand. Dip the extension in the glue and attach to your isolated lash
- Curved tweezers: use this to isolate the one targeted natural lash with the non dominant hand
- Mini Scissors: to cut your medical tape
- Tape: to hold the bottom lashes and patches down
- Gel patches: to hold down bottom lashes and mini treatment for under eye circles and puffiness
- Disposable mascara wands: used to comb through the lashes (must use different one every time for each individual client)

- Medical grade Adhesive (Glue): to bond extension to the natural lash
- Jade stone: this is where you will put your glue on, the stone keeps the drop of glue from drying for as long as possible
- Jade stone disposable covers: used to place over jade stone to save time and energy from cleaning jade stone. The cover can be thrown away when done
- Glue remover: to remove any unwanted lashes or glue
- Micro applicators: tiny brushes used to remove 1 lash extension at a time along with the remover
- Disposable flocked applicators: used to remove the lashes along with the remover
- Eyelash trays: trays that hold the eyelash extensions
- Makeup remover : eyelash extension friendly remover to remove makeup
- Primer: preps the lashes and removes any excess proteins and oils left on the lashes
- Acetone: removes dried up glue on the jade stone or tweezers
- Alcohol: disinfects tools
- Nano mister: allows for the adhesive to cure instantly without having to wait 24-48 hrs for lashes to dry
- Air blower or fan: creates air in order to reduce fumes from glue
- Emergency eye wash: in case of emergency, pour the complete bottle immediately into the affected eye in case glue gets in the eye

Chapter 4

Hair Growth Cycle and Anatomy of Eyelashes

In this chapter we will look at the anatomy of the eyelashes, to really understand the biology behind it and why certain things are the way they are. Our lashes protect against dust, particles, intense light etc. Lashes have their own growth speed and everyone's speed is different.

 The Eyes can have about maximum 200 lashes each in general. The lengths of the upper natural lashes, usually vary anywhere from 6-12 mm and lower lashes natural lengths are from 2-8 mm.

People can lose anywhere from 1-5 lashes a day. Lashes vary from fine to medium to thick and can be straight, crisscrossed, semi curved, very curved, going in every direction and curly etc. But your job, is to make the extensions look perfectly straight regardless of the natural direction of the lash.

We all have an Eyelash cycle 60-90 day hair cycle. Lashes are constantly falling and growing back. Here is how the cycle works;

-Anagen stage also known as baby hairs
-Catagen stage also known as teen hairs

-Telogen stage also known as adult hairs (hair that is about to shed)

Here is the cycle and how it works. Inside the dermis, under the telogen hair, there is an anagen hair waiting to come out. Once the the telogen has reached it's full growth, it then falls and the anagen grows out. The anagen hair then turns into catagen (best stage to put false lashes) and then the cycle repeats itself. Never put false lashes on an anagen hair, it will damage it, sometimes even cause permanent hair loss. An anagen hair is too weak and thin for eyelash extensions.

As you can see in the diagram below, after a telogen hair falls, the hair underneath grows out and the cycle repeats itself.

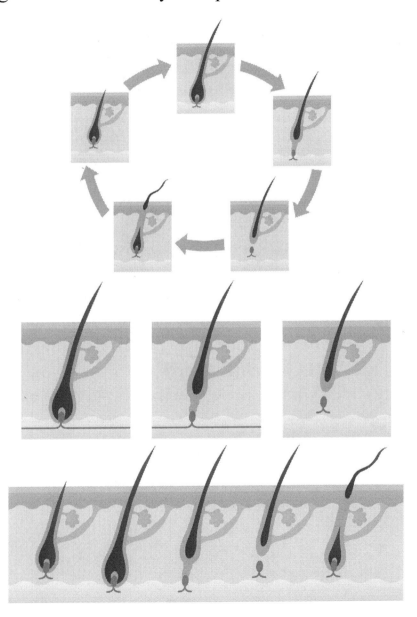

Chapter 5

Health & Safety

Here are some health and safety measures you will have to do in order to ensure the health and safety of the lashes!

- Discuss if the client has any eye problems, has had any recent surgery, takes medication, has allergies etc.
(Make sure the client has no allergies to any of the ingredients and products you will be using and have her sign a waiver form)
- Wait 3 months after a surgery or laser and 2 weeks after someone has permed or tinted their lashes. If at any time you are unsure, ask for a doctors note
- Client's eyes must be closed and stay closed the entire time
- Always offer clients good quality products
- Apply lashes one by one and choose the appropriate extensions for that client
- Apply the extensions 2mm away from the root of the eyelid, never touch the skin

Which Clients to Avoid

Clients with:

- Unhealthy skin around the eyes and/or redness, crusty lashes
- Client with infection (conjunctivitis, pharyngitis)
- Itchy eyes or allergies. Have them consult a pharmacist for an antihistamine since you cannot offer medical advice
- Cancer patients, undergoing chemo or any medical treatment, recent surgeries, any medical condition that you are not familiar with (doctor's note)
- People with weak eyelashes who are not good candidates. Avoid them or offer a growth serum. Rebook them for an appointment in several weeks. (Refer to chapter 8 for in depth home maintenance instructions and products)
- People who want an extreme look but are not eligible
- People who don't listen to your instructions or just charge them accordingly. Example; a client uses products that contain oil to clean her eyes at night. Her lashes don't last long because of this. If she comes back for a refill in 2 weeks but has hardly any lashes, you would charge her for a full set.

Client complaints

- It is normal to sometimes feel discomfort or irritation due to the fumes in some cases (depending on client's sensitivity, make sure the clients eyes are well closed throughout the entire process)
- Pain, itchiness or discomfort, can be caused by the extensions being

stuck together or too close to the skin

- Irritation days later can be caused by not allowing the glue to cure properly and vapour could still get into the eyes

Hygiene for the Technician

- Wash your hands properly, germs stay under nails and in between fingers and palms of hands. It is recommended to sing the complete happy birthday song while washing your hands for proper timing. You can also disinfect them with hand sanitizer afterwards
- Dress well and appropriate, nails maintained, some makeup, clean hair, good body odour etc.
- Mascara brushes, patches, applicators, lash extensions or glue used for previous client, should not be used on someone else

Disinfecting tools

Always disinfect your tweezers in between clients (have two sets of tweezers)

1- Place tweezers and jade stone in pure acetone to remove excess glue or use a disposable jade stone film

2- Wipe and soak in rubbing alcohol for 10 minutes

*Never drop your tweezers, dropping them could cause a misalignment and tweezers will break

Client Hygiene

Your clients need to keep their eyelash extensions clean (clients can develop Blepharitis due to poor eye hygiene). Blepharitis is a condition of the eyes that causes inflammation and possible infection of the eyelid due to a blocked eyelash follicle. Please educate your clients.

Some symptoms of Blepharitis are as follows:

-Burning Sensation
-White flaking on and between lashes
-Crusting on the eyelids
-Swollen eyes
-Itchiness
-Redness

Chapter 6

Structures, Eye Shapes and Styles

Sizes
7-11 mm is considered a natural look
12 mm is considered the transition from natural to dramatic
13-17 mm is considered dramatic

Basic Structures

The numbers used are only examples, any size can be used for these structures. Imagine that your client is lying down on her back with her head facing yours.

These examples are from the left eye to right eye. The left eye goes from outer to inner corner and the right eye demo starts from the inner to outer corner.

The eye needs to be separated in 3 or 4 depending on the technique you decide to use. The lines can be drawn on your patches until you are experienced enough to do it by eye.

A basic structure:	left eye 10-10-8	8-10-10 right eye
Advanced basic:	left eye 10-9-8-7	7-8-9-10 right eye
Basic cat eye structure:	left eye 14-12-10	10-12-14 right eye
Advanced cat eye:	left eye 12-11-10-9	9-10-11-12 right eye
Open eye structure:	left eye 10-12-10	10-12-10 right eye

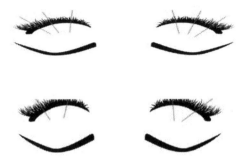

Eye shapes and Styles/Corrections

Almond eyes (universal shape)
Considered most desired shape

-Can do any style

Close set eyes

Distance between the eyes are smaller than the actual width of one eye

How to correct this:
-Apply the Cat eye structure
-Extensions should be longer and thicker in the outer corners of the eyes
-little extensions should be used in the inner corners of the eye

Wide set eyes
Opposite of close set

How to correct this:
-Extensions should be thicker in the inner corners of the eye
-little extensions should be used in the outer corners of the eye
-No cat eye

Monolid eyes
A single eyelid, eyes are usually small in nature

How to correct this:
-Use C-D-L curls they will open up the eye and give the illusion of an eye crease
-Add longer lashes in the centre of the lid (open eye structure)

Hooded eyes
Droopy skin, natural crease appears hidden

How to correct this:
Use C-D-L curls these curls will give the illusion of an eye crease and hide the droopy skin

Deep Set eyes
Pronounced eye arch, protruding eyebrow bone

How to correct this:
-Avoid C-D-L, these are too curly and could potentially touch the protruding bone
-Use same lengths along the eyelid example 10-10-8 | 8-10-10 (basic structure)

Protruding eyes
Eyelid appears to be bulging

How to correct this:
-Do not surpass 12 mm
-No C-D-L
-Use B to reduce bulging effect

Upturned eyes
Natural upward lift at outer corners of eyes

How to correct this:

-Avoid cat eye

Down turned eyes

Slight to visible droop at the outer corners

How to correct this:

-Do the basic cat eye example but with a twist (using any numbers in the following example) add 10-12-10-8 | 8-10-12-10 (start with smaller lengths in the outer corners to give an illusion that the corners of the eyes are lifted higher than they really are)

Chapter 7

Preparation, Application and Removal

The Preparation

- (For first time client) Discuss with your client what she would like and explain the process and rules
- Disinfect hands and tools (preferably in front of your client)
- Have the client lie on her back with her head towards you
- Remove any makeup on the eyes and/or any excess dirt and proteins on the eyelashes
- Apply patches to the bottom lashes to protect them (avoid touching the waterline) apply your medical tape to hold down the patches and cover the bottom lashes
- Tape could be applied to the upper eyelid if client has droopy skin
- Brush the lashes and begin

The Application

- Apply a tissue on client's forehead, since you will be resting your hands on the client's forehead throughout the procedure

- Choose the right extensions and prepare glue (shake the glue bottle and add a drop to your jade stone)
- With your non dominant hand, isolate a natural lash with your curved tweezers
- With your dominant hand, take your straight tweezers, grab an extension and dip the base 1/3 of the way into the glue
- Take that same extension and swipe it along the isolated lash and coat it with glue (swipe 3 times) 2mm away from the root and let go
- Repeat these steps by alternating from one eye to the next, try to do the same steps for each eye, do this until the lashes are completely full
- Use both tweezers to separate the lashes and verify that none are stuck together (crucial)
- Once you are satisfied, comb through the lashes
- Dry and cure the lashes with the help of your air blower and nano mister
- Remove the tape and patches making sure there is no glue or lashes stuck to it
- Voila! You have just completed a set of eyelash extensions

Refills

Same steps as the preparation section. After applying the patches and tape, clean and remove any unwanted extensions in order to have a clean start. Proceed with the remaining preparation and application steps.

How to Remove Lashes

- Apply the preparation steps as if you were going to do a set of eyelash extensions
- Clients eyes must remain closed the whole time, opening the eyes can really irritate the client
- Apply the remover
- Let it sit for 5-10 minutes
- Remove with flocked applicators and clean the lashes (lashes will slide right off)
- Remove the tape and patches (eyes must remain closed)
- Rinse eyes with a wet cotton pad
- Dry eyes
- Client can open her eyes

*Use the twist and peel method to remove a single extension from a natural lash. This is a process where you would grab the extension with the curved tweezer (non dominant hand) and the natural lash with the straight tweezer (dominant hand). Peel them apart. This is completely safe, as long as you're not pulling the lash out of the follicle.

Factors that can Affect the lifetime and health of lashes

- Incorrect bonding

- Mascara residue
- Extension applied on weak lashes
- Natural cycle (some people lose lashes faster than others)
- Too much or not enough glue
- Wrong extension size or thickness applied to the natural lash
- Home maintenance and 48 hour rule not being respected
- Two lashes or more glued together
- Rubbing eyes or pulling lashes

All of this can cause temporary to permanent damage. Having two or more lashes stuck together is dangerous. Aside from the fact that the client will feel a painful, tugging sensation, one lash could be growing faster than the other, causing the other lash to fall prematurely. This can cause trauma to the lash and permanent hair loss.

Chapter 8

Client Home Maintenance

These next steps are crucial for your clients. They must follow them in order to protect their natural lashes from damage, to maintain the lifetime of their lashes and to avoid developing eye infections.

#1 Makeup remover and/or cleanser

Client must have an eyelash friendly makeup remover and/or cleanser. Products with oil will ruin the bonding of lashes. Your clients need to keep their eyelash extensions clean otherwise they risk the chance of developing infections.

#2 A growth serum

This is obligatory for every client. It is what protects the natural lashes from the weight and damage that lash extensions might have over time and create a solid base for bonding. You can offer growth serums to clients who are not good candidates for lash extensions, for those with weak or damaged lashes, or women who want that dramatic look. Helps your lashes reach their full potential in length, fullness, thickness and darkness.

Also moisturizes and provides nutrients for the eyelashes, while protecting them from breakage.

Can also be worn without extensions.

*Beware of unknown online suppliers

#3 Coating sealers

The coating sealer protects against factors that will affect the life bondage of the extended lashes such as, climate, oil, moisture etc. Leaves a glossy finish to the lashes. Use his product every 3 days, can be used everyday. It is usually water washable

#4 mascara

For clients who still want to wear mascara or fill gaps before their scheduled refill.

How To Educate Your Clients

Clients need to be educated on maintenance and caring of their lashes. Once they leave your salon or studio, they will need to have precise instructions on how to care for their lashes and what not to do, to prolong the bonding life.

- No pulling on lashes
- Refills 2-4 weeks
- 48 hour rule (no wetting the lashes, no makeup, no tanning, no exercising, no vapour for 24-48 hours) unless you use the nano mister
- Avoid oil
- Use eyelash friendly products
- No mascaras (unless it's eyelash friendly) especially not waterproof
- No eyelash curlers unless it is a heated curler

Chapter 9

Marketing and Pricing

Here are 10 rules or tactics that will help you succeed in your eyelash extension business.

1-Research companies (your competition) in your area, see what they are charging.
In general:
Full set price: salon price; 100-150. Home services; 60-75
Refills: salon price; 50-75. Home services; 30-40

2-Find your target market (who are you trying to reach) and advertize to them by posting on social media; Facebook, twitter, instagram (speak to these people, add them, follow them, always give something back, give them information by starting a blog, Youtube channel, or writing articles).

3-Advertise in the paper or local adds

4-Make business cards, flyers, car magnets, put adds in pharmacies, salons, schools (universities). Trade with professionals, leave your cards in their salon and vice versa.

5-Start working in a salon to get experience and get to know the business. You can also do employees' lashes for half price or even free in order to advertise.

6-Putting adds in people's mailbox (the homes of your target market, a specific class of people).

7- Go to networking events.. network, network, network!

8-Word of mouth, always sell yourself, always mention what you do.

9-Wear eyelash extensions, women will 100% stop you and ask you about them, give them your business card at this point

10-Get insurance or have them sign a waiver form at their first appointment.

Congratulations on your decision to becoming an Eyelash Stylist!! Eyelash extensions are the hottest thing right now!

Please leave us an Amazon review for this book and let us know what you think.

Visit Julia Broderick's Youtube channel (BeautifulHealthyMom) for more beauty tips and beauty techniques!

https://www.youtube.com/user/beautifulhealthymom1

Watch Julia's eyelash extension video:

https://www.youtube.com/watch?v=gfP1t-d239E

Made in United States
Orlando, FL
01 October 2023

37475154R00022